Manuela Stoicescu

Side Effects Of Antiviral Hepatitis Treatment

Manuela Stoicescu

Side Effects Of Antiviral Hepatitis Treatment

Medication Risks Of The Currently Available Treatment Options

LAP LAMBERT Academic Publishing

Impressum / Imprint

Bibliografische Information der Deutschen Nationalbibliothek: Die Deutsche Nationalbibliothek verzeichnet diese Publikation in der Deutschen Nationalbibliografie; detaillierte bibliografische Daten sind im Internet über http://dnb.d-nb.de abrufbar.

Alle in diesem Buch genannten Marken und Produktnamen unterliegen warenzeichen-, marken- oder patentrechtlichem Schutz bzw. sind Warenzeichen oder eingetragene Warenzeichen der jeweiligen Inhaber. Die Wiedergabe von Marken, Produktnamen, Gebrauchsnamen, Handelsnamen, Warenbezeichnungen u.s.w. in diesem Werk berechtigt auch ohne besondere Kennzeichnung nicht zu der Annahme, dass solche Namen im Sinne der Warenzeichen- und Markenschutzgesetzgebung als frei zu betrachten wären und daher von jedermann benutzt werden dürften.

Bibliographic information published by the Deutsche Nationalbibliothek: The Deutsche Nationalbibliothek lists this publication in the Deutsche Nationalbibliografie; detailed bibliographic data are available in the Internet at http://dnb.d-nb.de.

Any brand names and product names mentioned in this book are subject to trademark, brand or patent protection and are trademarks or registered trademarks of their respective holders. The use of brand names, product names, common names, trade names, product descriptions etc. even without a particular marking in this works is in no way to be construed to mean that such names may be regarded as unrestricted in respect of trademark and brand protection legislation and could thus be used by anyone.

Coverbild / Cover image: www.ingimage.com

Verlag / Publisher:
LAP LAMBERT Academic Publishing
ist ein Imprint der / is a trademark of
OmniScriptum GmbH & Co. KG
Heinrich-Böcking-Str. 6-8, 66121 Saarbrücken, Deutschland / Germany
Email: info@lap-publishing.com

Herstellung: siehe letzte Seite /
Printed at: see last page
ISBN: 978-3-659-47428-6

Copyright © 2013 OmniScriptum GmbH & Co. KG
Alle Rechte vorbehalten. / All rights reserved. Saarbrücken 2013

Table of contents

Introduction..2
Therapy with interferon...4
Therapy with ribavarin..7
The mains side effects of therapy with interferon and ribavarin........................8
1. The decrease of the immunity of the body – leucopenia........................8
2. Moderate and severe anemia..10
3. Thrombocytopenia..12
4. Central pancitopenia- myelosuppresion..26
5. Severe allergic reactions at drugs..28
6. Dermatologic side effects...29
7. Immune disorders...29
8. Acute and sub acute renal failure..32
9. Nausea, vomiting, joint pain and loss hair..34
10. Asthenia, loss of muscular strength..34
11. Carcinogenic risk (breast carcinoma)...35
Conclusions..40
References...41

Side effects of antiviral hepatitis treatment

Manuela Stoicescu
Consultant Internal Medicine, PhD, assistant Professor
University of Oradea, Faculty of Medicine and Pharmacy
Medical Disciplines Department
Romania

Introduction

At this moment the therapy of the patients with chronic viral B or C hepatitis remain yet a problem open for research. The efforts doctors all over the world must be orientated in this direction because the solution for these patients is far from being found.

During the period in which therapy with Pegylat @ Interferon and Ribavarin was discovered everybody believed that this represented the solution for chronic viral B and C hepatitis with the view of removing the virus from the body thanks to this protocol. But after the standard protocols of therapy where applied in medical practice it was observed that a small proportion of the patients responded very well to the therapy a second portion had an incomplete response to the therapy and many others have no responsible to this therapeutic protocol.

I personally, in my medical practice, during this period of time approximately 15 years, in reality I have not seen a single clinical case in which therapy with Pegylat @ Interferon alone or in association with Ribavarin has eliminated virus B or virus C from the body, there appeared to be a partial amelioration of the disease as the analyzed blood test showed a decrease in the level of cytolyses liver enzymes (ASAT, ALAT) glutamate aminotransferase and oxalate aminotransferase-and decreased viremia (the virus B or C remained in the body of the patient) but this has a price very important side effects we can't neglect and a significant number of patients did not tolerate this complete protocol of therapy and this must to be stopped or reduced for a shorter period of time compared to the standard protocols administered and currently used in the medical practice.

After this was believe that the patients that did not respond well from therapy with Pegylat @ Interferon if they followed a new scheme of therapy with Ribavarin in the end virus B or C on the eliminated with success from the body but this new therapy is done with only one agent as several other agent may have cumulative side effects for the patient, with decreased quality of life and increased risk of mortality by others affections they induce. Of course these side effects are more severe and serious if the duration of the therapy is longer and the dosages of medication are higher and when both preparations are associates in double therapy.

Considering these side effects, it should be honestly considered by doctors all over the world administering this treatment, who are confronted every day in the medical practice with these situations to write about the side effects of therapy with Interferon and Ribavarin because only in this mode can a final right decision be taken with regards to categories of patients who are unfortunate to come into contact with virus B or C in one moment of life and in this moment we can establish exactly what the problem might be.

We must have the courage to recognized the problem of these patients are not solved yet and we do not have to give false hope to our patients with this actual schemes and protocols of treatment which are far from ideal, more than that followed by serious side effects, this should serve as an alarm signal.

Also comparative studies about the medium rate of survey and the quality of life of the patients with active chronic hepatitis virus B or C positive who effected protocols of therapy and who did not follow any protocol of therapy was not conducted seriously. This evidence could give surprising results which are not in favor of actual schemes of therapy.

I decided to write about this topic of research, because I want to help these patients who suffer from consecutive and numerous clinical observations from my medical practice every day confronted frequently with these clinical cases as an internal medicine doctor.

I believe with strong opinion that this therapeutics protocols must be reevaluated in the medical practice and also other doctors must be encourage to relate other clinical observations from their medical practice about the side effects of therapy with Interferon and Ribavarin which must be substantiated and publish. The balance between the risks and benefits I believe should be seriously reevaluated.

Personally, in the future, I believe that these actual protocols will be substitute with other therapeutic schemes and the maximum benefit will be represented by prophylaxis, also large programs to inform the people, especially the young about the possibilities of transmission and the modalities of contaminations with virus B and C these infections could be more responsibly prevented hence avoiding all therapy schemes.

I want to thank all the people who agree with the clinical presentation I will follow to present. Also I want to encourage other doctors to publish their clinical observations and opinions about this very interesting topic of clinical research.

Also I want to thank you Sir Dmitrii Ghimisli, Acquisition Editor, LAP LAMBERT Academic Publishing is a trademark of: AV Akademikerverlag GmbH & Co. KG, Heinrich-Böcking-Str. 6-8, 66121, Saarbrücken, Germany.for the invitation to write this chapter of the book after his interest was manifested in my research "The risks of therapy with Interferon and Ribavarin", without this book it will not exist.

Therapy with interferon

The Interferon@ and β, makes part from categories of modify of biologic response. The utilization of Interferon in the medical practice in therapy of the patients with chronic viral hepatitis with respect to the criteria's of selection of the patients represent a direction relatively new in which a lot of hope and expectations were placed when this therapy was first discovered.

The role of this drug was to eliminate the hepatitis B virus from the body; concretization to eliminate circulating viral markers: AgHBe, AND-VHB, polymerase (AND p), clearance of the AgHBs, normalization of the liver biochemical parameters and also to prevent liver carcinoma.

The criteria's for selection was: the existence of a active chronic hepatitis without sign of the liver cirrhosis, the existence of the viral markers of diagnosis AgHBs, AgHBe, Ac anti HBe, AND-VHB, IgM anti HBs, Ag-preS1 and the system of Ag/AcHBe. The level of liver enzymes must to be twice increasing comparative with the normal range and decrease level of viral replication (AND -VHB under 200pg/ml).

The contraindications were: advance liver cirrhosis decompensate parenchimatous and vascular, other severe associated disease such as: cardiac's, renal failure, lower immunity of the body, depressives syndromes, thyroidal disease, hyper sensibility of Interferon, asymptomatic patient with AgHbs+.

The side effects recognized were: somatic - pseudo grippe syndrome, mialgias, headache, asthenia, anorexia, digestive disorders, vertigo and loss of hair. Neuoropsihycs - insomnia, disturbance of concentration, irritability, depression, psychosis. Biological: leucopenia, thrombocytopenia, susceptibility to infections (bacterial spontaneous peritonitis), autoimmune manifestation (thyroidal). The types of responses were individualized in four categories:

1. Complete response

The disparities between AND-VHB and AND-p, which are maintain after the therapy is stopped and sero-conversion in HBe system and HBs system

2. Incomplete response

Sustain inhibition of replication VHB which is maintained after the therapy is stopped, sero-conversion in the system HBe but with persistence of AgHBs

3. Transitor response.

Disparities of the markers of replication but only in period of therapy.

4. Missing response (No response)

The ideal scope of this therapy was the elimination of the markers of viral

replication and sero-conversion in the system HBs. There were possibilities to optimize the therapy:
- By increase the dosages, prolonged the cures of treatment, repeated the protocols or
- Association with acyclovir, ARA-AMP, IL2, Lamivudin
- Association IFN 3MU 3 times /week with ganciclovir (3X1g/day)

The true is all this esperance of the protocol of therapy with Interferon wasn't confirmed in the medical practice. More than that with the price of a serious secondary side effects and we cannot neglected the reality is that our patients remain continue chronic with the AgHbs with different forms of chronic hepatitis: easy, medium and severe types in the presence of other association risks factors and with the continue risk to develop in one moment the carcinoma of the liver.

Also they continue to remain a source of infection and contamination and transmission the virus at other innocent persons. Another important aspect is the increase grade of irresponsibility of this persons with positive virus B or C, who don't declare this , don't protect himself and also no protect other peoples around in transmission of virus B or C. These peoples must be more correct responsabilisation about the disease.

Interferon-alpha (IFN-alpha) has been extensively explored for its efficacy in various disease conditions and is currently used as a standard treatment in several of these. Its use is accompanied by a wide variety of possible side effects [1] These side-effects may hamper reaching and maintaining the dose needed for maximal therapeutic effect while their occurrence can outweigh clinical benefit of IFN-alpha treatment. [1] This review addresses the toxicity profile of IFN-alpha, the presumed path physiology of the different side effects and the strategies to handle these.

Adverse effects due to IFN-alpha have been described in almost every organ system. Many side-effects are clearly dose-dependent. Taken together, occurrence of flu-like symptoms, hematological toxicity, elevated transaminases, nausea, fatigue, and psychiatric sequel are the most frequently encountered. Although insight in the mechanisms accounting for IFN-alpha-related toxicities has improved in recent years, much remains to be elucidated. Guidelines on the management of this untoward sequel are mostly based on clinical experience, while many side-effects can only be adequately handled by dose adjustment or cessation of treatment [1] Further research on the mechanisms underlying both therapeutic effects and adverse events is warranted. Hopefully, this will lead to better identification of those patients who are likely to benefit from treatment without experiencing severe toxicities.[1]

Therapy with ribavarin

Ribavarina – guanosinic analog is active on viruses AND and ARN, inhibit the guanil transferase, metiltransferase and polymerize r ARN and increase the inhibitor effect of macrophages on viral replication. The administration is oral and believed to have good tolerance. The dosages are between 1000-1200mg/day time by 4-6 months .Is indicated in chronic C hepatitis in absence of a response during therapy with Interferon after three months, alone or in association with interferon. The therapeutic trials are in the course of evaluation. Ribavarin monotherapy is not effective for the treatment of a chronic hepatitis C virus infection and should not be used alone for this.

The principal side effects evaluated is hemolytic anemia depends on dosages, affirmatively reversible after it is stopped, I personally saw cases of breast carcinoma after association therapy with Interferon and Ribavarin. After stopping this therapy the patient did not recover from anemia without the right therapy being implemented. The primary clinical toxicity of Ribavarin is hemolytic anemia. The anemia associated with Ribavarin therapy may result in worsening of cardiac disease and lead to fatal and nonfatal myocardial infarctions. Patients with history of significant or unstable cardiac disease should not be treated with Ribavarin. [See Warnings and Precautions [5, 2] Adverse Reactions 6, 1, and Dosage and administration [2, 3].

Significant teratogenic and /or embryocardial effects have been demonstrated in all animal species exposed to Ribavarin. In addition, Ribavarin has a multiple dose half-life of 12 days and it may persist in non-plasma compartments for as long 6 months. Therefore, Ribavarin, including Ribavarin tablets, is contraindicated in women who are pregnant and in the male partners of women who are pregnant. Extreme care must be taken to avoid pregnancy during therapy and for 6 months after completion of therapy in both female patients and in female partners of male patients who are taking Ribavarin therapy. At least two reliable forms of effective contraception must be utilized during treatment and during the 6 month post treatment follow- up period.[see Contraindication[4] Warnings and precautions[5,1], and Use is Specific Populations[8,1].

Chronic hepatitis C is a disease of the liver caused by the hepatitis C virus. The disease can be serious and even fatal. Approximately 25% of patients with chronic hepatitis C will develop cirrhosis and some of these patients will develop cancer of the liver or liver failure.

Presently the disease is treated with a combination of alpha interferon or peginterferon (antiviral and immune stimulating drugs) and ribavirin (an antiviral drug). Alpha interferon is given by injection three times a week whereas peginterferon is given by injection only once a week. Ribavirin is given as a tablet by mouth twice a day. The combination therapy is given for 6 to months. About half of the patients given these medications will receive a lasting benefit and many patients do not respond well to the combination therapy.

The mains side effects of therapy with Interferon and ribavarin
1. The decrease of the immunity of the body - leucopenia

An important side effect of therapy with Interferon and Ribavarin is decreased immunity of the body and higher risks of infections with different localizations in the body. We must not forget that these patients have a low immunity because the presence of the virus B or C in the body. Also they can have an initial leucopenia because it is possible for the phenomena of hipersplenism to exist and the leucopenia decreases after the therapy with Interferon and Ribavarin. If the number of leucocytes is normal before therapy, the level of leucocytes will decrease after this therapy and can develop severe values. I observed clinical cases in my medical practice that developed a very severe leucopenia after following therapy with Interferon and Ribavarin, for example 2000/mm3 or 1000/mm3 level and after that developed severe infections complicated by septicemia which was difficult to treat with three antibiotics in association with a therapeutic scheme.

I will follow by presenting the clinical case of a patient 52 years old who was diagnosis with chronic active viral hepatitis after laboratory examination with increase viremia level and the biopsy of the liver confirmed the diagnosis of active chronic viral hepatitis.

The patient followed the therapy with Interferon with @Interferon 3MU 3 times/ week during three weeks. After three weeks of therapy he developed chills, fever 40,5 °C, sweating and the level of leucocytes become 1000/mm3, the level of thrombocytes was 150 000 and red cells= 3 millions.

The patient followed therapy with leucocytes mass i.v. 4UI. After was recoated hem cultures and came positive with Clostridium dificille therapy was started with three antibiotics together twice/day, but under therapy with this associations of antibiotics the fever still persisted approximately 2 weeks such as sub febricities 37,8 ° C and only after three weeks of therapy with 3 combinations of antibiotics did the fever decrease completely and the level of leucocytes increased to level 4000/mm3 after 4UI i.v. leucocytes masses. The diagnosis at the moment was: Severe leucopenia, Septicemia with Clostridium difficile. Active chronic hepatitis virus C positive. This was the result of decrease the immunity of the body in context of side effect after therapy with Interferon

Another important observation are the higher rate of association of infections with virus C positive and diabetes mellitus, and also the diabetes mellitus diseases decrease the immunity of the body and the risk of infections and septicemia are higher in these conditions.

A total of 3,882 Japanese patients [2] with chronic hepatitis C were given interferon (IFN) alone or combination therapy of IFN and ribavirin. Two hundred sixty-one (7.7%) patients stopped IFN therapy due to the adverse events after initiation of IFN therapy alone. About a half of patients with side effect discontinued the IFN regimen due to owing to general fatigue, psychiatric disorder, thrombocytopenia, and leucopenia. On the other hand, 82 (16.2%) patients stopped combination therapy of IFN and ribavirin due to the adverse events. We should carefully observe the patients treated with IFN. If patients treated with IFN have IFN-related adverse effects, we should stop IFN therapy or reduce the dose of IFN.

Meds Facts [3] provides MD-approved analysis to help both patients and physicians accurately research and assess the risk-reward trade off for more than 20,000 different pharmaceutical products. Between January 2004 and October 2012, 3 individuals taking Interferon alfa-2B recombinant (Interferon alfa-2B) reported leukopenia to the FDA. A total of 16 Interferon alfa-2B recombinant (Interferon alfa-2B) drug adverse event reaction reports were made with the FDA during this time period. Often the FDA only receives reports of the most critical and severe cases; these numbers may therefore under represent the complication rate of the medication.

2. Moderate and severe anemia

Anemia moderate or severe forms represent another important complication after therapy with Interferon and Ribavarin. This is a common side effect of treatment for chronic hepatitis C virus (HCV) infection, due to red blood cell destruction (hemolytic anemia) caused by ribavirin and bone marrow suppression related to interferon.

Erythropoietin (Procrit) and other erythropoiesis-stimulating agents (ESAs) that boost red blood cell production may be used to manage anemia. Reducing the dose of ribavirin is also done to control anemia, but this may increase the risk of post-treatment relapse, and therefore decrease the likelihood of achieving sustained response.

The severe clinical cases I saw in my medical practice with the level of red cells 1 million UI/mm3 , the value of Hemoglobin was 4g/dl , Ht=18% with put the problem to excluded a bleeding, which wasn't confirmed and which necessitated transfusion of a blood iso group isoRh to correct the anemia.

The truth is that after stopping the protocol of the therapy with Interferon and Ribavarin to the patients who develop a severe anemic syndrome as a secondary reaction (side effects) at therapy , frequent transfusion of blood iso-group- isoRh for correcting the anemia is necessary , if the value of hemoglobin was under 8g/dl and this protocol was not as reversible as the doctors believed, after the of therapy is stopped, initially it is contrary sustain it and adequate therapy must to be given with iron drugs and folic acid for a long period of time to reverse the anemia and it is not in all cases this becomes completely solved, the existing situation when the anemia continues to persist also after the scheme therapy is followed which, produces dizziness in the patient , asthenia, a dynamic and permanent third sensation.

I present the clinical case of a patient age 48 years old who after following the protocol of therapy with Interferon and Ribavarin for active chronic hepatitis developed a very severe anemia with the level of Hemoglobin=6g/dl, red blood cell level=2,8 million/mm3, Ht=28% and she had to stop the therapy for this reason. She had to follow blood transfusion with blood iso group, isoRh 4UI to review the level of Hemoglobin at 10g/dl. Of course in the first instance was excluded the diagnosis of upper bleeding or bleeding in other sites but this was not confirmed and no other cause of anemia was found after complete laboratory tests were performed and was interpreted as side effects after this therapy.

Among the hematologic abnormalities associated with combination therapy, anemia is probably the most significant, as it can reduce patients' health-related quality of life and may be the main determinant of fatigue.[4] A pooled analysis of data from three large trials comparing pegylated interferon (peginterferon) with nonpegylated interferon determined that worsening of fatigue scores was a significant predictor of treatment discontinuation.[5] Interruption and premature discontinuation of antiviral therapy decreases the efficacy of antiviral therapy. In large multicenter clinical trials of combination therapy for HCV infection, dose reduction for anemia occurred in up to 23% of patients.[6,7]

Discontinuation was uncommon in these trials, but the rate of discontinuation is higher outside of clinical trials. In one study that evaluated "real world" patients, anemia was the leading cause of premature discontinuation of combination therapy, accounting for 36% of all discontinuations (ie, in 8.8% of all patients).[8]Significant anemia (ie, hemoglobin < 10 g/dL) has been observed in up to 9% to 13% of patients receiving combination therapy with interferon and ribavirin. 1 Moderate anemia (hemoglobin < 11 g/dL) may be seen in 30%. [9] The mean maximal decrease in hemoglobin can be as high as 3.1 g/dL and 3.7 g/dL with nonpegylated and pegylated interferon, respectively, in combination with ribavirin.2,8 The hemoglobin generally reaches its lowest level within the first 4 to 8 weeks of therapy, plateauing thereafter and returning to baseline values after treatment discontinuation.

3. Thrombocytopenia

Thrombocytopenia represents another side effect of therapy with Interferon and Ribavarin. The decrease number of platelets can be easy, moderate and severe. Also in the cases with severe thrombocytopenia appeared non palpable thrombocytopenic puerperal and bleeding syndrome. In this situation is necessary transfusion of platelets mass for correct the thrombocytopenia.

IFN-α has been proposed to induce thrombocytopenia mainly by inhibiting proliferation and maturation of megakaryocytes.[10,13] Autoimmune-based destruction of platelets[14,16] and capillary sequestration have also been proposed as causes of IFN-α–induced thrombocytopenia. [15,17].

I follow on to present the clinical case of a patient 42 years old who was diagnosed with active chronic hepatitis with virus B positive , who after following the protocol therapy with Interferon and Ribavarin developed a menoragia-menstruation period was prolonged to 14 days, with hipermenoreea, clots and dysmenorrheal . Initially was suspected the diagnosis of uterine fibroid which was confirmed after Para clinical examination (abdominal eco, abdominal CT, endo vaginal eco) and gynecological consult.

The blood test was highlighted a very sever thrombocytopenia with value = 20

000/mm3 which necessitated administrating the platelets masses repeated 4UIi.v. and haemostatic medication to stop the bleeding. I want to mention that the patient had the level of platelets in normal range (280 000/mm3) before the patient started the protocol of therapy with Interferon and Ribavarin.

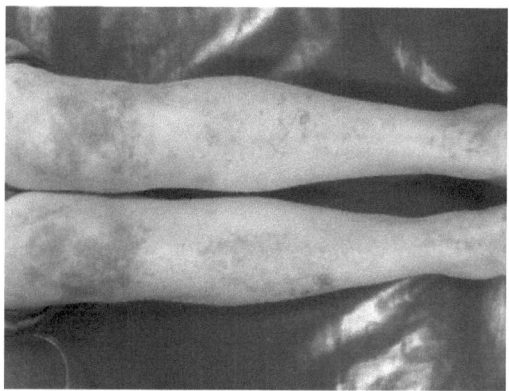

Figure1. Purpura on the legs

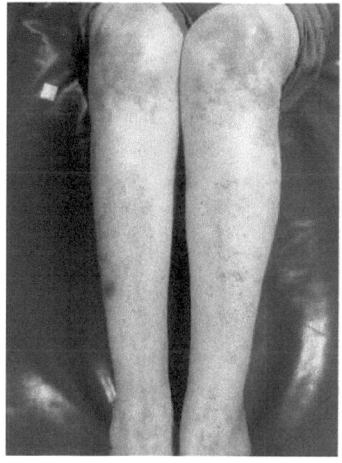 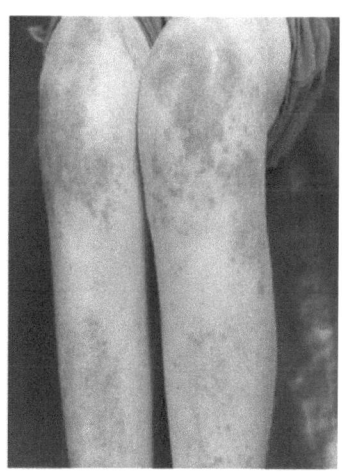

Figure 2 Purpura on the legs   **Figure 3 Purpura on the legs**

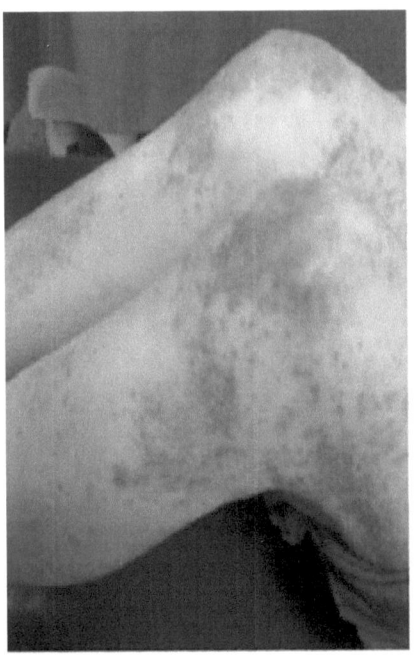

Figure4 Purpura on the legs

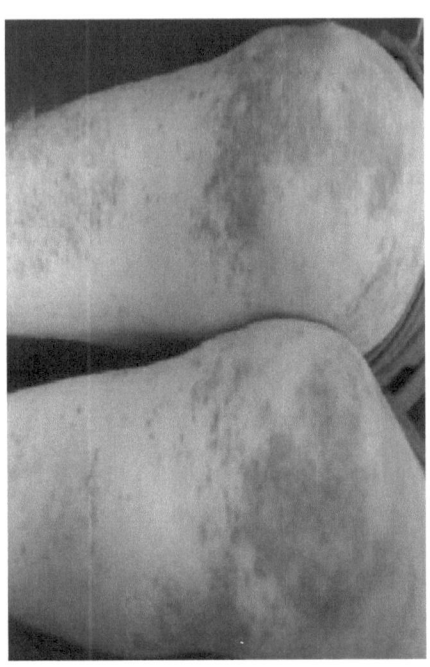

Figure5 Purpura on the knee

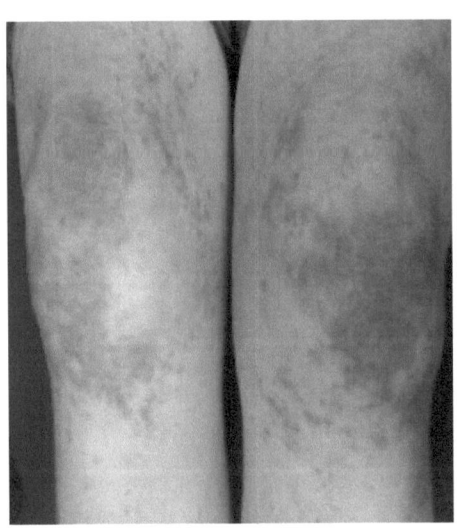

Figure6 Purpura on the knee

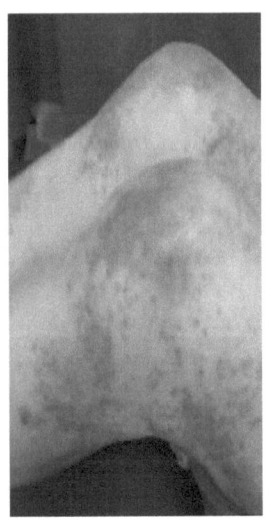

Figure7Purpura on the knee

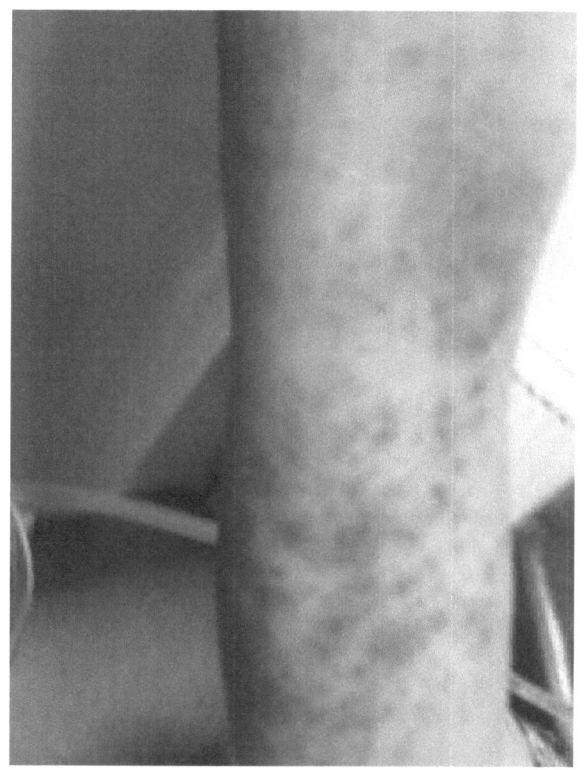

Figure 8 Purpura on the arm

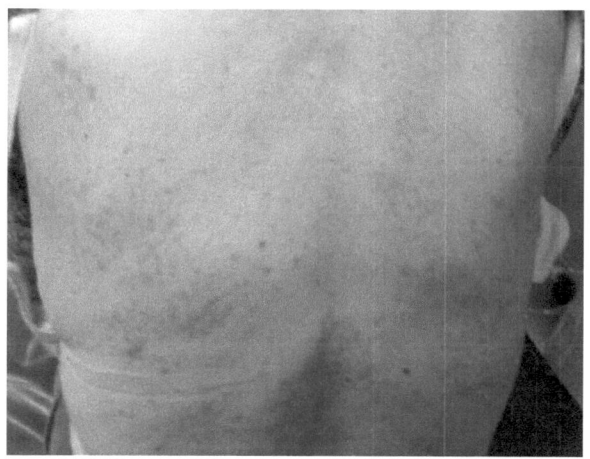

Figure 9. Purpura on the posterior chest

The next clinical case from my medical practice evidenced the same side effects - the thrombocytopenia and possible carcinogenic risk. I present the clinical case of a man 52 years old who came for a consultation because he felt asthenia, a dynamic sensation that causes loss in force and he can't work for a long period of time for this reason, everything began approximately six months ago. One week ago there appeared jaundice and a brown color of his urine shown in the images below: **(Figures10 - Figures16)**

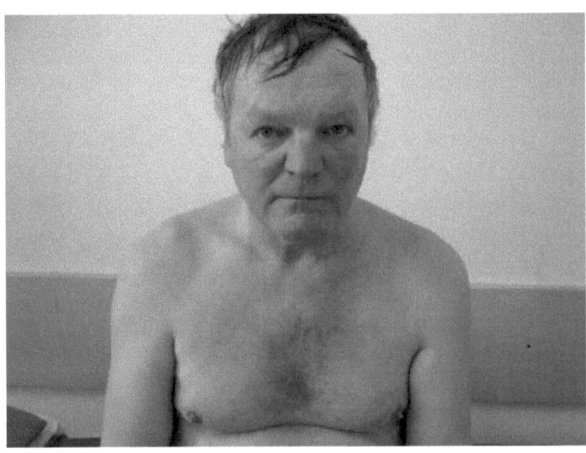

Figure10. Jaundice at the scleras and skin

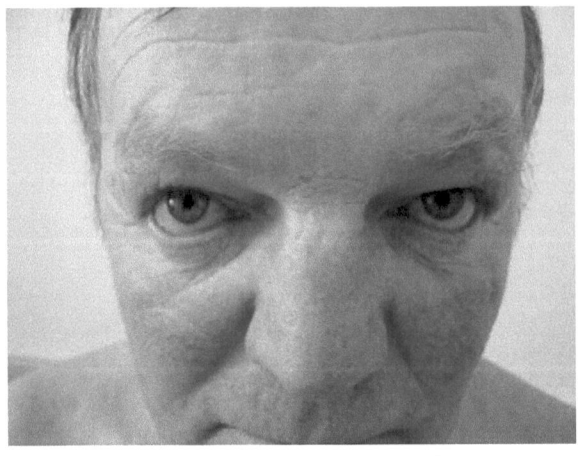

Figure11. Jaundice of the scleras

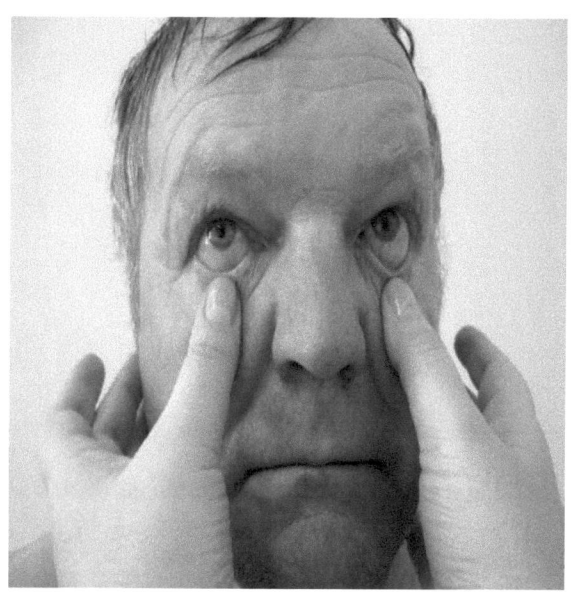

Figure12. Objective examination of the scleras revealed jaundice

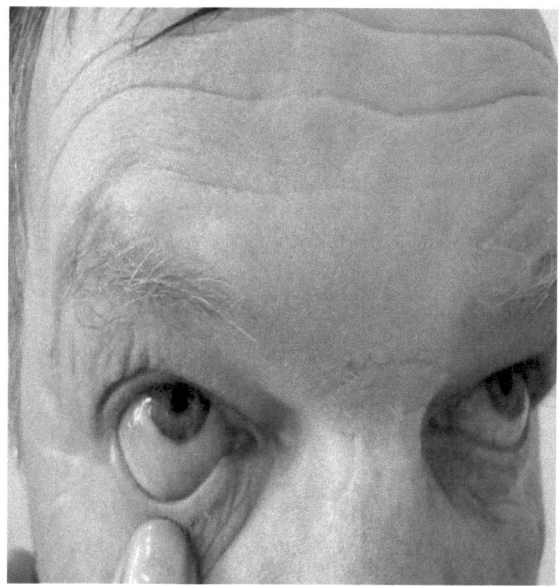

Figure13. Objective examination of the scleras-jaundice

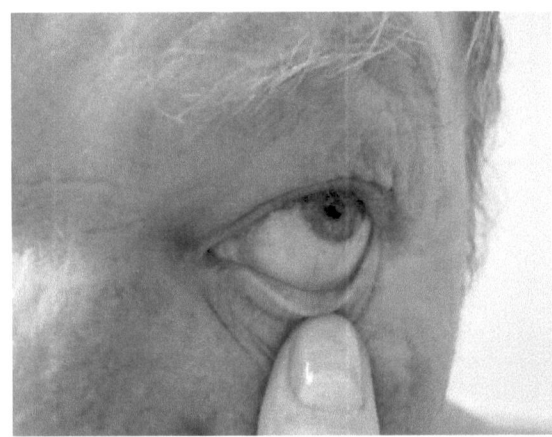

Figure14. Objective examination of the sclera-jaundice

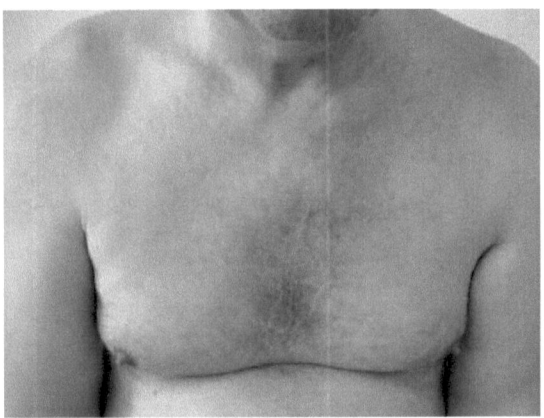

Figure15. Jaundice of the skin

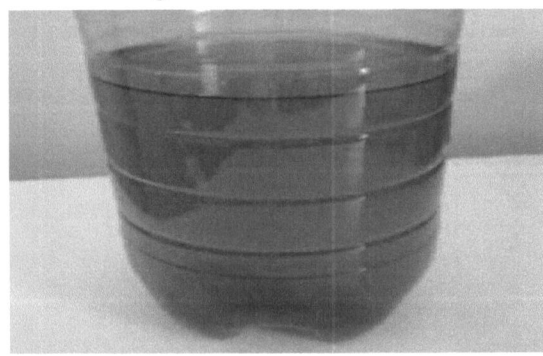

Figure16. Choluric urine

At the objective examination red palms or liver palms was present also **(Figure 17)**, one tattoo like a heart on the left arm **(Figure18)**, clubbed fingers **(Figures 19-22)**, aspect of the coated tongue **(Figure 23)**, jaundice also appeared under the tongue **(Figure 24)** shown in the images below.

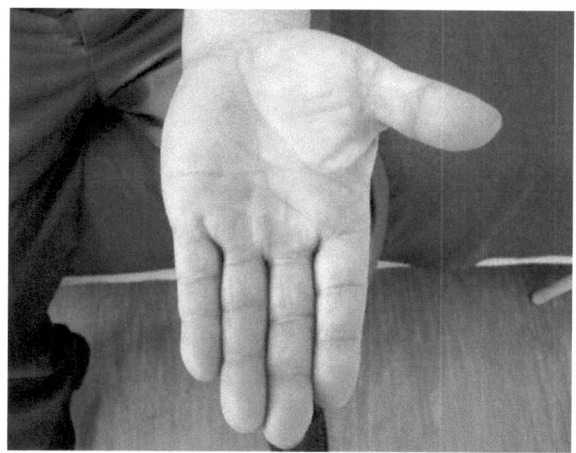

Figure17. Red palm – Liver palm

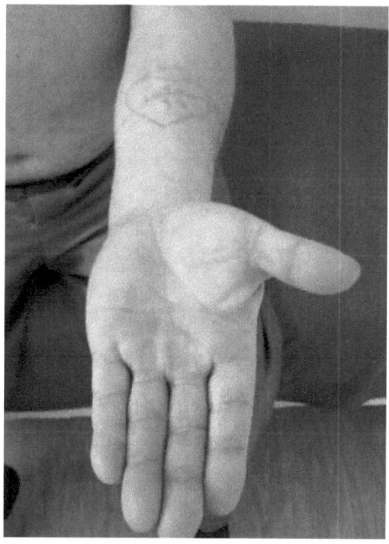

Figure18. Tattoo and liver palm

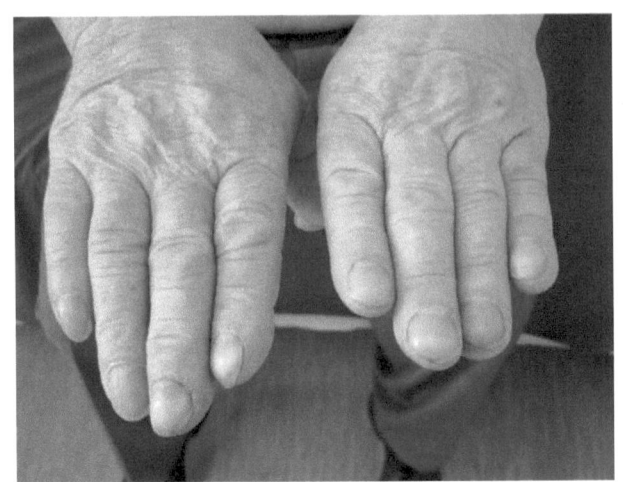

Figure19. Clubbed Fingers

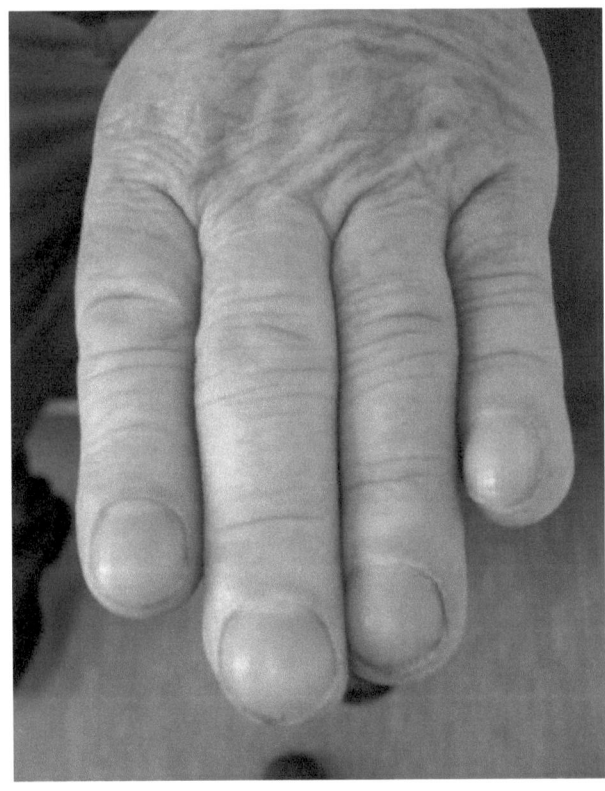

Figure20. Clubbed Fingers

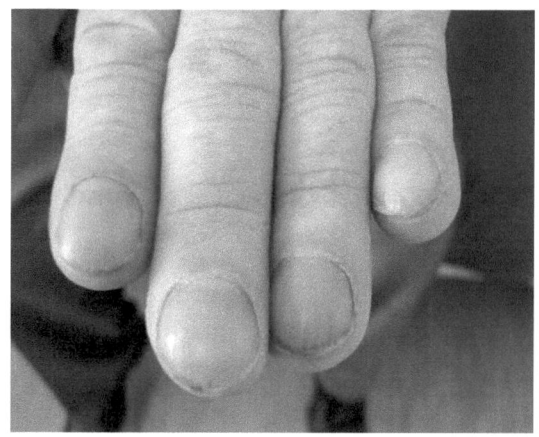

Figure21. Clubbed Fingers

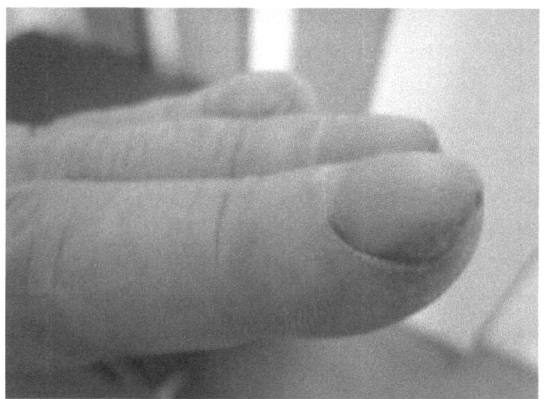

Figure22. Clubbed Fingers

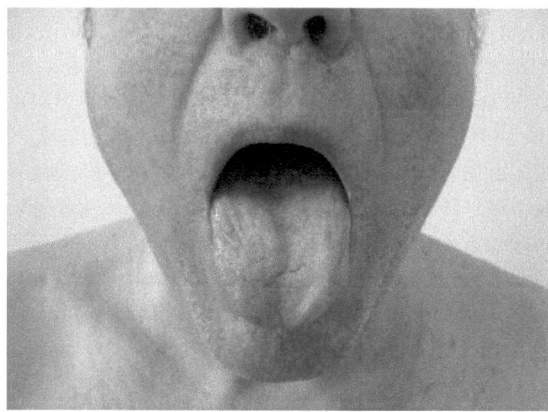

Figure 23 Appearance of the tongue – coated tongue

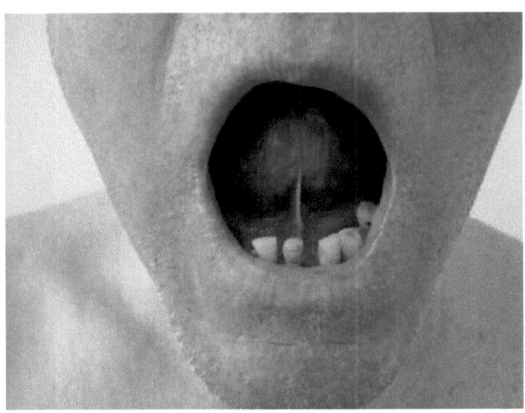

Figure 24 Appearance under the tongue revealed jaundice

The blood tests revealed: ASAT=238UI/l, ALAT=302UI/l, total bilirubin=3,2mg/dl, indirect bilirubin=2,8mg/dl, gammaGT=101UI/l, alkaline phosphatase=76UI/l,bleedingtime=2,3sec,coagulation time =1,8sec, cholinesterase= 1213UI,redbloodcells=6,200000/mm3,leukocite=6000/mm3 ,platelets =200000/mm3 ,VSH=4mm1h-8mm2h,fibrinogen=250 mg%, glycemia=16mg/dl, cholesterol= 150mg/dl,triglyceride=128mg/dl,urine summary=Ubg positive, urinary sediment = normal, Atc antiVHC positive, viremia=7 000 000 millions UI. In this moment the diagnosis was established, active chronic viral C hepatitis positive. The risk factor for contamination was considered to be the moment when the patient performed the tattoo at the left arm. Abdominal eco confirmed hepatomegaly with increased echogenity and normal portal vein=11mm.After that the patient performed needle hepatic biopsy which showed the histopathology diagnosis of "piece meal necrosis". For this reason the patient follow the therapy protocol with α Interferon 6MU 3X/week and Ribavarin 1000mg/day six weeks with decreased viremia=1 000 000IU/ml, normalization of liver enzymes and persisted Anti-HCV positive. After that follow diet and liver protect medication with Silimarin 3x1 pills/day and Essential 3x1 pills-day. After this protocol of therapy the patient presented a purpura eruption on the legs **(Figure25)** with a sudden testicular bleeding we had to administer haemostatic drugs by perfusion to stop the bleeding such as Vitamin K and adrenostazin ampoules and the blood test revealed a very severe thrombocytopenia 50 000/mm3 which imposed administration of platelets mass in perfusion 4UI and after was performed a testicular echo **(Figure 26)** a tumor of the right testicle was discovered. After the surgical intervention the histopathology examinations confirmed a testicular adenocarcinoma. **(Figure 27 A-F)**

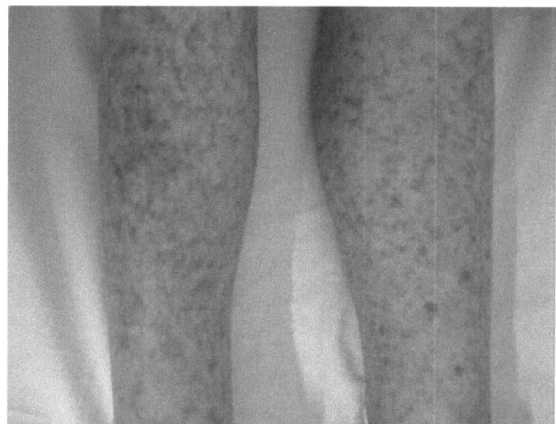

Figure25. Purpura in remission of the legs.

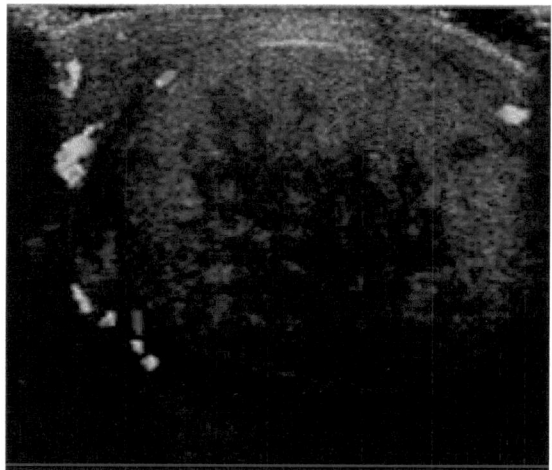

Figure 26 Right testicular tumor ultrasonography image

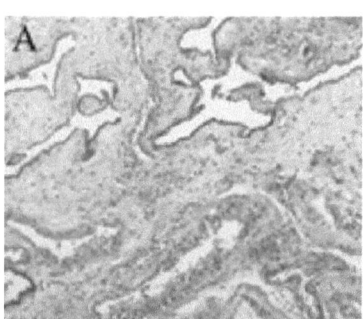
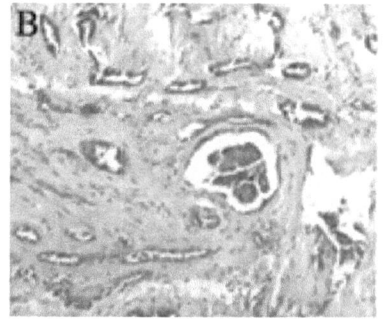

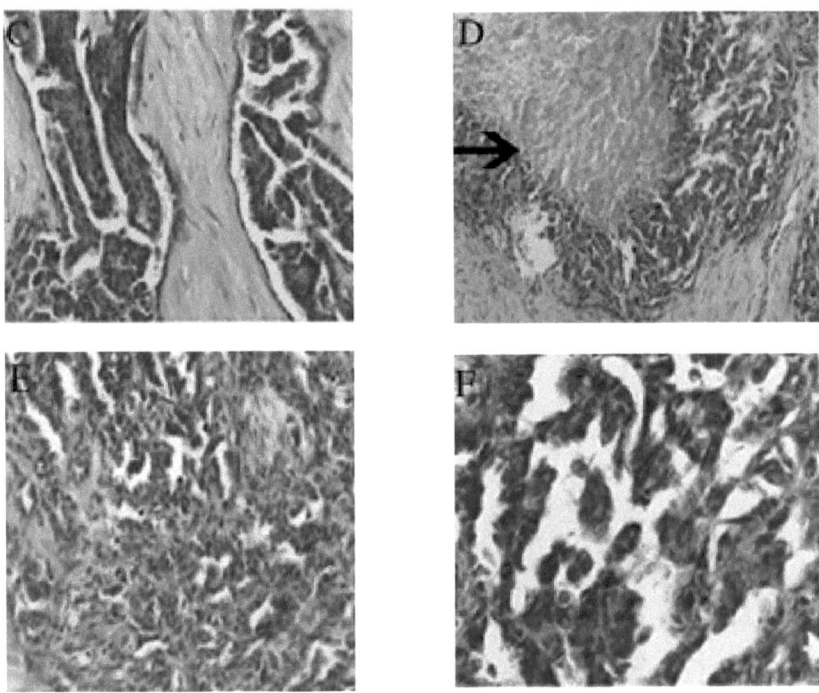

Figure27 (A-E) Testicular adenocarcinoma – histhopathological examination

Morphological change of the tumor. A, The remaining normal rete testis tissue was present in the peripheral area of the tumor. B, The area comprising irregular tubules with highly collagenized stroma represented adenomatous hyperplasia of the rete testis. C, In the distended tubules, the cells formed apparent papillary patterns. D, The apparent necrosis (black arrow) was present in the papillary structure. E, The area was composed of irregular small tubules and complicated papillary structures with little collagenized stroma. F, The cells had marked cellular atypia with dark staining chromatin and conspicuous nucleoli.

In conclusion a severe thrombocytopenia 50 000/mm3 appeared like side effects after protocol of therapy with Interferon and Ribavarin to develop a testicular bleeding and revealed a testicular adenocarcinoma.

A decrease in platelet count also may be observed in patients who are receiving interferons, and such decreases are more prominent with the peginterferons. A decrease in platelet count also may be observed in patients who are receiving interferon, and such decreases are more prominent with the peginterferons .The decrease is caused primarily by a reversible bone marrow suppression, although autoimmune related thrombocytopenia may also occur. The concurrent use of ribavirin may blunt the thrombocytopenic effect of interferon as a result of reactive platelets. With peginterferons, the platelet count decreases gradually over 8 weeks, stabilizing thereafter and returning to baseline values within 4 weeks of stopping therapy. Bleeding complications as a result of thrombocytopenia are uncommon but possible. [6, 7]

In randomized clinical trials of the peginterferons,the rate of dose reduction attributed to thrombocytopenia ranged from 3% to 6%.[6,7] However, most patients in clinical trials are carefully selected, and these trials excluded patients with more advanced liver disease. Patients with cirrhosis may have baseline thrombocytopenia due to hipersplenism from portal hypertension, and these patients may develop more significant decreases in platelet counts owing to bone marrow suppression during therapy. For these patients, an alternative approach to dose modification would be beneficial to avoid dose reduction or discontinuation, both of which reduce the chance of SVR.

Early, unencouraging results with interleukin-11

Data are even more limited on the use of growth factors for the management of interferon-related thrombocytopenia than for the management of interferon related anemia and neutropenia. Oprelvekin, or recombinant human interleukin-11, is approved for use in cancer patients receiving chemotherapy to enhance platelet production. It also may be useful as adjuvant therapy in HCV-infected patients receiving combination therapy. Oprelvekin was evaluated in an open-label study of 13 HCV-infected patients undergoing therapy with interferon (3 MU three times per week) and ribavirin (1,000 to 1,200 mg/d) for 48 weeks.[18] All patients had low baseline platelet counts (< 100,000 cells/mm3). Oprelvekin was given concurrently at a dose of 50 mg/kg subcutaneously three times per week.

The researchers noted improvement in platelet counts: the mean count at 2 weeks was higher than the baseline count (98,600 vs 73,600 cells/mm3; $P < .05$). The main side effect was fluid retention, which was noted in all patients, with 10 of 13 patients requiring diuretic therapy. Given this side-effect profile in patients with HCV-related cirrhosis, there currently is not much enthusiasm for oprelvekin's use. Newer growth factors with more promising safety and efficacy profiles are in development.

4. Central pancitopenia- myelosuppresion

Another dangerous side effects after protocol of therapy with Interferon and Ribavarin are the decrease of the levels of all figurate elements: anemia, leucopenia and thrombocytopenia with develop an acute bone marrow insufficiency (failure) confirmed after sternal puncture and decrease the level of reticulocites. The most frequent and numerous cases are acute leukemia.

Granulocytes, platelets, and red blood cell counts are commonly decreased during treatment. These are usually mild if normal counts are present initially, but can be dose limiting in the presence of low counts, for example in patients with hypersplenism. Patients may be predisposed to infections. The mechanism of granulocytopenia is unknown, but inhibition of cell release from the bone marrow has been suggested.

Follow to present the clinical case of a patient 58 years old that was diagnosed with active chronic hepatitis with virus C positive. After follow the protocol of therapy with alfa Interferon the patient develops sudden after three weeks of therapy: leucopenia=3000/mm3, anemia= 2 millions/mm3, thrombocytopenia=80 000/mm3, reticulocites level=0, 8‰ and for this reason the therapy must to be stopped. The sterna puncture confirmed the acute leukemia.

Interferon treatment is known to cause hematologic changes such as thrombocytopenia, anemia and granulocytopenia or combinations thereof. Patients followed by alpha interferon treatment developed even more severe pancytopenia and aplasia. Case reports of two patients who received treatment with alpha interferon 2a are reported here. Both patients were previously treated with IFN administration. Patient one developed life-threatening bone marrow hypoplasia and aplasia after interferon treatment and died. Patient two showed similar but less severe changes in bone marrow, i.e. thrombocytopenia, mild leukopenia and anemia. The clinical course of both patients was followed by routine peripheral blood tests and bone marrow biopsies and permits some reflection on the pathogenesis of marrow hypoplasia. Myelosuppressive effects of interferon treatment are discussed, cytokine actions and potential additional influences of herpesvirus infections.

Hepatitis-associated aplastic anemia is a common syndrome in patients with bone marrow failure. However, hepatitis-associated aplastic anemia is an immune-mediated disease that does not appear to be caused by any of the known hepatitis viruses including hepatitis C virus.

I report the case of a 52-year-old man who developed severe aplastic anemia during treatment with pegylated interferon alpha 2a for chronic hepatitis C virus infection. He presented with generalized purpura and bruising, as well as pallor of the skin and mucous membranes. His blood tests showed pancytopenia. He underwent allogeneic bone marrow transplantation after completing two courses of immunosuppressive therapy with antithymocyte globulin and cyclosporin A.

The combination of a specific environmental precipitant represented by the hepatitis C virus infection, an altered metabolic detoxification pathway due to treatment with pegylated interferon alpha 2a and a facilitating genetic background such as polymorphism in metabolic detoxification pathways and specific human leukocyte antigen genes possibly conspired synergistically in the development of aplastic anemia (Figure 28) in this patient. The case clearly shows that the causative role of pegylated interferon alpha 2a in the development of aplastic anemia must not be ignored.

Figure28. Bone marrow- aplastic anemia

5. Severe allergic reactions at drugs

Another very interesting phenomenon happened after protocol of therapy with Interferon and Ribavarin is the modification of the immunity of the body by the development of the antibodies which determine the apparition of the allergic reaction after drugs given to the patient who wasn't allergic before and these drugs could be administered without any problem before the protocol of therapy with these medications.

In this context I follow to exemplify this with a clinical case of a patient 42 years old who was diagnosed with active chronic hepatitis with the level of viremia and biopsy of the liver with histopathology examination revealed "piece meal necrosis".

Before the protocol of therapy with Interferon and Ribavarin the patient had a right basal pneumonia for which he performed the allergic test for Penicillin G and it was negative after that the patient follow the therapy with Penicillin G 2X1 000 000UI i.m./day ten days with complete resorbtion of the pneumonia and perfect tolerance to this therapy.

After the patient used the protocol of therapy with Interferon and Ribavarin it decreased only the levels of liver enzymes, viremia, the virus C still persisted and the patient developed again clinical symptoms of left basal pneumonia with which therapy with Penicillin G could be used again. Again the test of allergy to Penicillin was performed and at the time of the test the patient developed suddenly a strong allergic reaction (anaphylactic shock) to which adrenaline in dilution i.v. must be administrated immediately, HHC i.v. and O2 by mask to save the patient's life, and of course after this unhappy event she could not follow therapy with Penicillin G.

I want to mention that by carefully was made again the test of allergy at Penicillin G but this could not be repeated in consideration that was tested before and after direct administration the patient could develop sudden death.

Another observation is that the response after haemostatic therapy is modified (diminish) in therapy of upper bleeding after protocol of therapy with Interferon and Ribavarin, comparative with the patient who didn't use this therapy and increase the rate of mortality by upper bleeding. It is evident that the therapy modifies the reaction of the body to the administration to other drugs.

The upper bleedings are more difficult to stop and therapy with haemostatic drugs (the period of bleeding are longer in this situation) compared with the prompt response to the haemostatic therapy which did not follow the protocol of therapy with Interferon and Ribavarin

6. Dermatologic side effects

A variety of rashes including erythema multiform have been noted. Pruritus can be troublesome. Mild hair loss is relatively common but is reversible. Local erythema is common. Psoriasis can develop de novo, or be aggravated, and is usually difficult to treat.

7. Immune disorders

Interferon has important immunomodulatory properties. Non-organ-specific antibody titers may increase, and indeed may be associated with autoimmune thyroiditis, hypothyroidism, and hyperthyroidism. [19-23] Other autoimmune endocrine diseases have been induced, but thyroid disease is particularly important.

[24] Thyroid disorders have been reported in 2.5-20 percent of patients. This may not be reversible after stopping therapy, unless therapy is stopped early, and long-term thyroid replacement may be required. [25-28] It is possible that underlying thyroid disease is more common in chronic hepatitis C infection.

An aggravation of the chronic hepatitis may occur. Patients may be genetically predisposed to this complication and can be recognized by prior autoantibody measurement and HLA haplo typing. An exacerbation of psoriasis may be part of this syndrome. Discontinuation may be required, particularly for hyperthyroidism, unless transient hyperthyroidism followed by hypothyroidism is recognizable. Autoimmune hepatitis usually necessitates discontinuation of therapy. Interferon may promote the development of lupus erytematosous systemic.

I am reporting the clinical case of a young woman patient 38 years old who after was diagnosed with active chronic hepatitis with virus C positive and followed the protocol of therapy with Interferon and Ribavarin she developed a systemic vasculitis with a lupus like syndrome. The aspect of the faces of the patient appeared after protocol of therapy with Interferon and Ribavarin and are shown in the images bellow: **(Figure29a-d)**

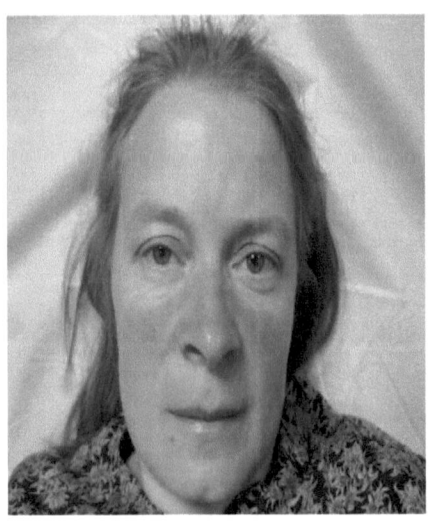 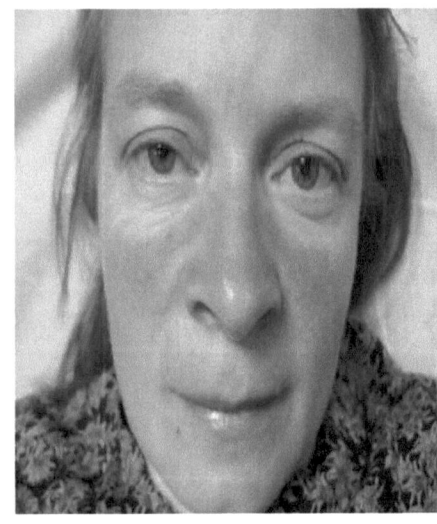

Figure29a Face in lupus   **Figure29b Face in lupus**

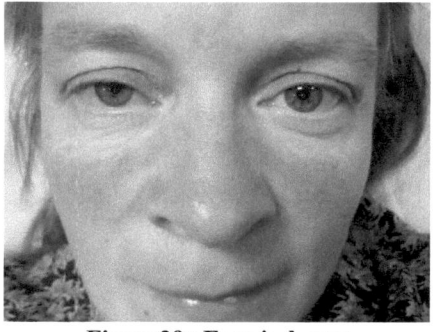 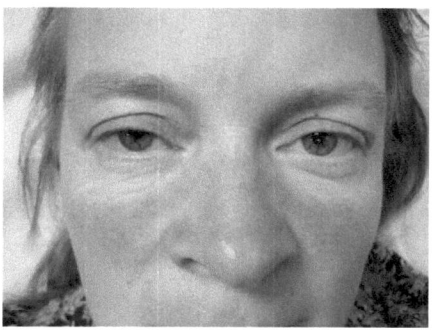

Figure29c Face in lupus   **Figure29d Face in lupus**

Near image   **Near image**

The patient presented chills, fever 39°C, purpura eruption of the legs, joint pain and swollen of the inter fingers joints of the hands in the morning shown in the image below **(Figure30)**.

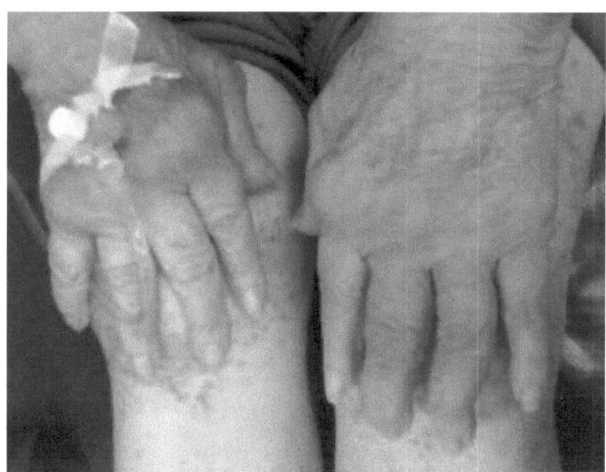

Figure30 Aspect of the both hands with swollen of inter phalange joints

The laboratory test confirmed the diagnosis of lupus erytematosous systemic this autoimmune disease by Autoantibody anti ADN double catena positive and LE cells positive and biopsy of the skin purpura relieved a leucocitoclastic vasculitis secondary in context of this autoimmune disease.

8. Acute and sub acute renal failure

The patients with chronic hepatitis virus B or virus C positive is possible to have a systemic vasculitis in the context of the disease without clinical manifestations (subclinical) unknown and with secondary nephropathy in this context with minimal nephritic syndrome manifested with isolated proteinuria, isolated hematuria or proteinuria and hematuria identify after summary urine examination was performed. If the patient had this result with nephritic syndrome after urine examination before she start the therapy with Interferon and Ribavarin for active chronic hepatitis with virus C or B positive, the patient has risk to develop after the protocol therapy sub acute or acute renal failure with severe evolution of the patient with rapid progressive azotes retention syndrome to necessary dialysis for the patients.

I present the clinical case of a patient age 48 years old who was hospitalized for the diagnosis of active chronic hepatitis with virus B positive with increase value of liver enzymes (TGO=248UI/l, TGP=342UI/l, Gama GT=121, indirect bilirubin=2,32,total bilirubin=3mg/dl, viremia=6 millions unites, Atc antiHCV+, liver biopsy with histopathology examination confirmed active chronic hepatitis , summary of the urine – Urobilinogen positive, proteinuria+, in rest normal and the value of urea=32mg/dl, creatinine=0,9mg/dl. After the patient follow the protocol of therapy with Interferon and Ribavarin presented the apparition of a palpable purpura at the level of inferior legs shown in the images below: **(Figure31)**

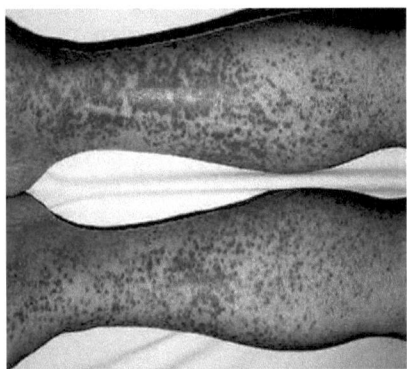

Figure31 Palpable purpuric rash at the lower limbs

And the nephritic syndrome was accented: proteinuria =30mg/dl, hematuria=20g/dl. The skin biopsy confirmed the diagnosis of systemic vasculitis (poliarteritis nodosa) shown in the image below:

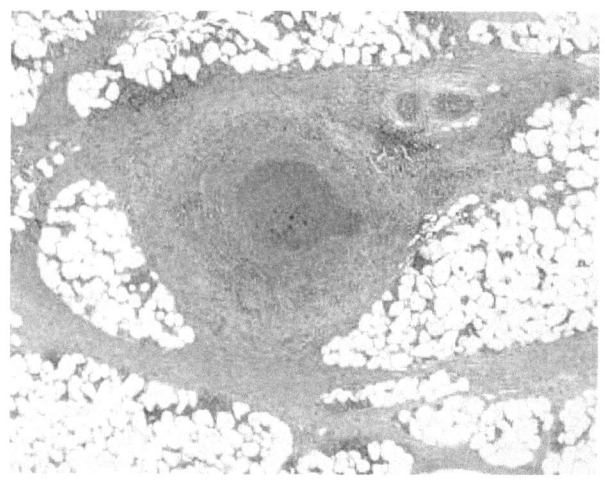

Figure32 The histopathological examination polyarteritis nodosa
Stain: hematoxylin and eosin.
Magnification:×40.

After the skin biopsy was performed the result confirmed safe diagnosis of polyarteritis nodosa. The histopathological examination **(Figure32)** with fibrinoid necrosis of the vessel wall with surrounding perivascular lymphocytic infiltrates, polyarteritis nodosa was confirmed as the safe diagnosis.

After that the patient developed a syndrome of progressive azotized retention uremia with increase level of creatinemia+5,08mg/dl and urea=402mf/dl with oligo-anuria so an acute renal failure in context of systemic vasculitis with secondary nephropathies hence an imposition of dialysis for the normalization of the azotized parameters.

Histopathological examination after kidney biopsy revealed sub acute glomerulonephritis.

9. Nausea, vomiting, joint pain and loss hair

Another side effect after administration of therapy with interferon and Ribavarin are: nausea, vomiting, loss of hair (side effect like after chemotherapy) and pain of the joints.

I present the clinical case of a patient 48 years old with active chronic hepatitis with virus C positive. Who after following the protocol of therapy with interferon and Ribavarin appeared to have nausea, repeated vomiting, joint pain and loss of hair.

The patient was completely investigated: all lab test amylasemia, amylasuria, upper endoscopy, abdominal echo, abdominal CT, colonoscopy, X-ray of empty, but everything was within normal limits except leucopenia=3000UI/mm3. So in conclusion any other causes of nausea and vomiting were not found. Only in the context of side effects after protocol of therapy with Interferon and Ribavarin can these symptoms be explained.

10. Asthenia, loss of muscular strength

All the patients after following therapeutic protocols with Interferon and Ribavarin suffered from asthenia and the loss of muscular strength. Because I observed these symptoms for all the patients I decided to follow the level of muscular enzymes CPK-MM (iso enzyme MM) and it was increased in all the cases. These suggested that there appeared a myositis after therapy with Interferon and Ribavarin. After this observation I decided to make muscular biopsy and the result confirmed myositis and also the immunologic test and antibody anti Mi2 was positive.

The conclusions are that after therapy with Interferon and Ribavarin appeared as side effect myositis which was manifested clinically with asthenia, a dynamic, loss of muscular strength and increased amounts of the supplementary levels of TGP not in context of active chronic hepatitis and also in the context of myositis.

More than that this polymyositis it is possible to be in the neoplazic context-paraneoplazic myositis syndrome and a cancer is possible to be situated in the stomach, colon and other organs in the body.

Dermatomyositis is frequently associated with cancer (lung, ovarian, colon etc.), this variation being a paraneoplasic syndrome, which may appear in the years to come to form a malignity. Chest X-ray images of the anterior-posterior view of a patient with dermatomyositis, which shows lung cancer with a peripheral starting point. Colonoscopy performed for one patient with dermatomyositis which shows adenocarcinoma of the colon.

Dermatomyosistis is an autoimmune disease with concurrent skin damage. Besides shawl sign there is the appearance of hypopigmented areas alternating with areas of hyper pigmentation, erythema, skin atrophy, teleangiectasis. These elements are defined poikilodermical, which can also be associated with dermatomiosytis, or other autoimmune disease may be autoimmune. It occurs is chronic forms, while Gottron papules appear in acute forms.

11. Carcinogenic risk (breast carcinoma)

The main objective of this clinical case presentation is to attract attention to the risk of therapy with interferon and ribavarin. I present the clinical case of a woman patient 44 years old, which came to consultation for asthenia, after following a diet for weight loss. The objective examination was within normal limits except the presence of the hepatomegaly at 1, 5 cm under the last rib, with regular border, increase consistence, regular surface, without pain in time of palpation. The laboratory examination showed: ALT=48UI/l, ALP=56UI/l, total bilirubin=1,8 mg/dL, indirect bilirubin=1,5mg/dL, direct(conjugated) bilirubin=0,3 mg/dL, Gamma GT=58IU/L, FA=36UI/L, serum protein=7.2g/100ml, serum protein electrophoresis albumin=28% α1=4% α2=6% β=10% γ=21%, serum immunoglobulin levels: IgG=720 mg/100 ml, IgM =96 g/100 ml, IgA=90mg/100ml, TS=1,2s, TC=1,4s. After I performed viral markers appeared Anti-HCV positive, Hepatitis B virus (HBV) negative, Anti-mitochondrial antibodies negative, viremia=5 000 000IU/ml. In this moment was established the diagnosis active chronic virally C hepatitis positive.

Abdominal eco confirmed hepatomegaly with increased echogenity and normal portal vein=11mm.After that the patient performed needle hepatic biopsy which showed the histopathology diagnosis of "piece meal necrosis". **(Figure33).**

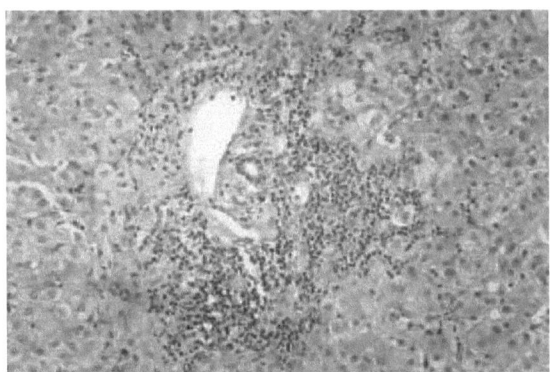

Figure33. Histopathology examination of liver - HE stain - Piece meal necrosis

It is important to note the discordance between the level of the liver enzymes (ALT=48UI/l, ALP=56UI/l) no very increase and the very severe active lesions, at the histopathology examination after needle biopsy of the liver, fulminate necrotic liver disease with "piece meal necrosis". The levels of liver enzyme no was at double level but because the result after needle liver biopsy was so severe and viremia at so increase values, the patient started therapy with α interferon. After this result the patient followed the standard protocol of therapy with α Interferon 6MU 3X/week three month but without response after therapy. The level of liver enzymes remained at the same value, Anti-HCV stayed positive, only viremia decrease to 3 000 000IU/ml level. For this reason the patient follow the therapy protocol with α Interferon 6MU 3X/week and Ribavarin 1000mg/day six weeks with decreased viremia= 1 000 000IU/ml, normalization of liver enzymes and persisted Anti-HCV positive. After that he followed a diet and liver protect medication with Silimarin 3x1 pills/day and Essential 3x1 pills-day.

In approximately 6 month after following the standard protocol with α Interferon and Ribavarin the patient presented appearance of a tumor formation 2,

5/3, 5 cm with irregular border, hard, with low mobility at the level of left breast which later was confirmed after performing mammography **(Figure34a and 2b)**, breast eco Doppler **(Figure35)** and needle breast biopsy with histopathology examination as a breast carcinoma **(Figure36).**

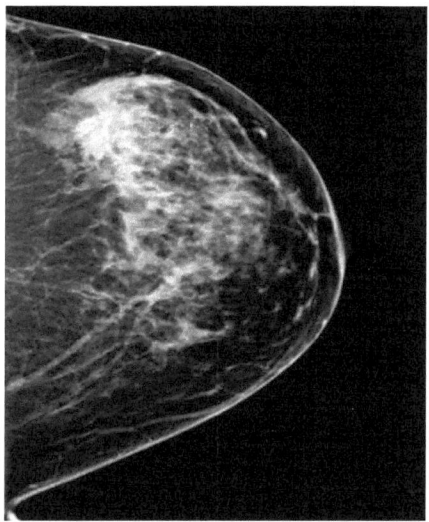

Figure 34a Mammography of left breast

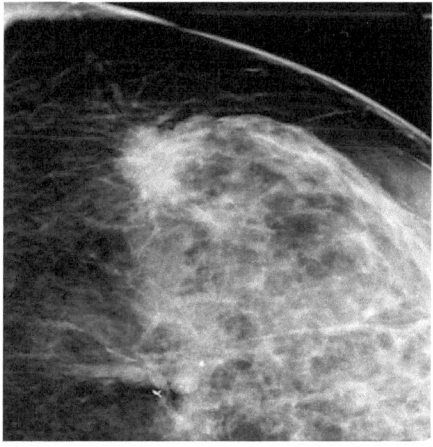

Figure 34b Mammography of left breast
Irregular tumor formation

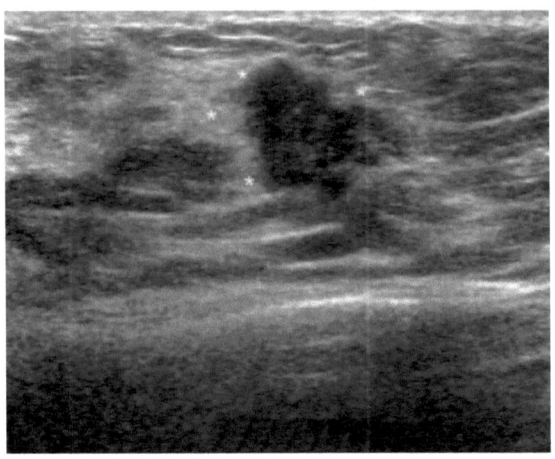

Figure 35 Breast echo Doppler– irregular tumor formation with increase vascular flux at the Doppler examination

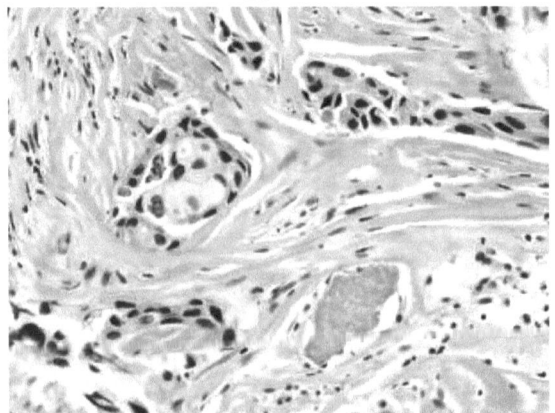

Figure36. Histopathology examination HE stain Breast invasive scirhous carcinoma

The patient had performed Halsted surgical intervention with tumor formation resection and lymph nodes extirpation of left axial side, radiotherapy and chemotherapy with favorable evolution. I mentioned that the patient did not present per heredity line cases of carcinoma of the breast and she performed a screening mammography **(Figure 37)** before she discovered that she was virus C positive and started the therapy with interferon and she recovered.

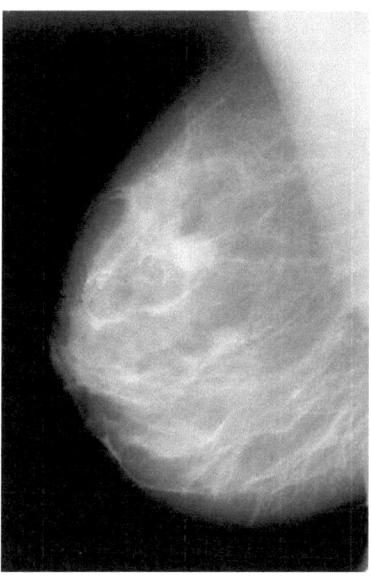

Figure 37 Normal mammography

Another clinical case from my medical practice revealed a women 66 years old who after was diagnosis with active chronic hepatitis with virus C positive and follow the standard protocol of therapy with Interferon and Ribavarin develop this red eruption on the skin at the right breast shown in the images below like an eczema – red and itching. **(Figure38a-c)**

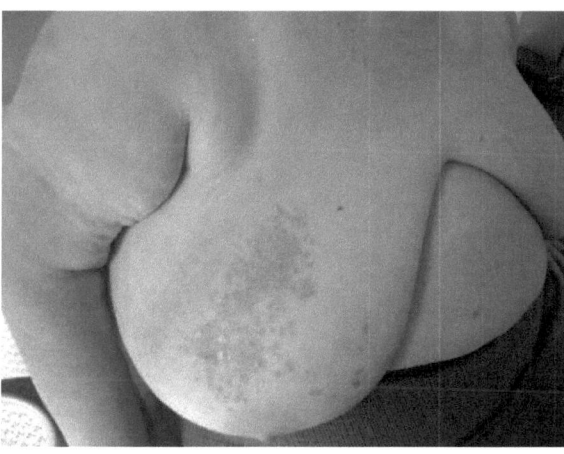

Figure 38a Red eruption on the skin - right breast

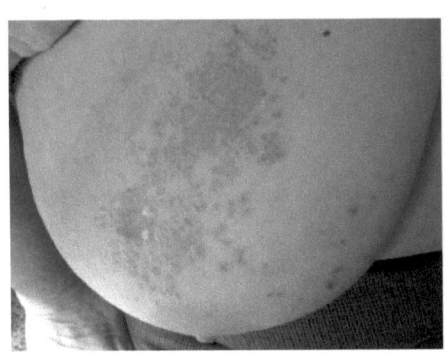 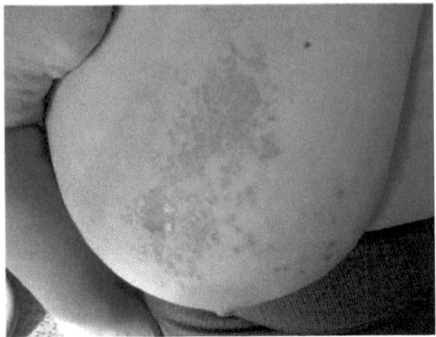

Figure38b Red eruption -right breast   Figure 38c Red eruption - right breast

In the first instance this patients went for a dermatological consultation where diagnosis was psoriasis eczema of the right breast and started a topical therapy with hydrocortisone cream but without any effect to the eruption, this persist the with the same macroscopic aspect after three weeks with this therapy. For this reason a biopsy was performed and revealed unexpected carcinoma of the breast. The patient follow right mastectomy and right axillaries lymph nodes resection (Halsted surgical intervention). The histopathology examination confirmed the breast invasive scirhous carcinoma.

Conclusions

1. I consider that at this moment we did not know all side effects of therapy with Interferon and Ribavarin in the scheme of chronic active hepatitis with virus B and C positive.

2. In our medical practice unexpected side effects are possible to appear any time and sometimes we must interrupt the protocol of therapy for this reason personalized to individual patient.

3. The associations with other disease make the problem more difficult.

4. It is sure that this therapy changes the immunity of the body with severe allergic reactions after different medications used after this protocol and we must be careful to test our patient so they do not develop unexpected anaphylactic shock after medications.

5. Autoimmune diseases could appear such as lupus erytematosous systemic, rheumatoid arthritis, dermatomyositis, systemic vasculitis.

6. We can't ignore the possible risk of cancer and also aplasia of the bone marrow with risk of different forms of leukemia.

7. I think with strong opinion that this actual therapy must to be reevaluated with seriousness and to take in consideration the risk and benefit.

8. In the future other drugs will replace this actual standard protocol of therapy.

References

1. **Pharm World Sci 2005 Dec. 27(6):423-31.** Side effects of interferon-alpha therapy. **Sleijfer S, Bannik M, Van Gool AR, Kruit WH, Stoter G.** Source Department of Medical Oncology, Erasmus University Medical Center-Daniel den Hoed Cancer Center, P.O. Box 5201, 3008, Rotterdam, AE, The Netherlands.

2. **Nihon Rinsho.** 2006 Jul; 64(7):1363-7.[Side effects of interferon therapy for chronic hepatitis C].[Article in Japanese].**AraseY** SourceDepartment of Gastroenterology, Toranomon Hospital.

3. **MedsFacts Meta-Analysis** covering adverse side effect reports of Interferon alfa-2B recombinant (Interferon alfa-2B) patients who developed leokopenia.

4. **Martin LM, Younossi ZM, Price L, et al.** The impact of ribavirininduced anemia on health-related quality of life. Hepatology 2001; 34(suppl):600A. Abstract.

5. **Bernstein D, Kleinman L, Barker CM, Revicki DA, Green J.** Relationship of health-related quality of life to treatment adherence and sustained response in chronic hepatitis C patients. Hepatology 2002; 35:704–708.

6. **Manns MP, McHutchison JG, Gordon SC, et al.** Peginterferon alfa-2b plus ribavirin compared with interferon alfa-2b plus ribavirin for initial treatment of chronic hepatitis C: a randomised trial. Lancet 2001; 358:958–965.

7. **Fried MW, Shiffman ML, Reddy KR, et al.** Peginterferon alfa-2a plus ribavirin for chronic hepatitis C virus infection. N Engl J Med 2002; 347:975–982.

8. **Gaeta GB, Precone DF, Felaco FM, et al.** Premature discontinuation of interferon plus ribavirin for adverse effects: a multicentre survey in 'real world' patients with

chronic hepatitis C. Aliment Pharmacol Ther 2002; 16:1633–1639.

9.**Kenilworth, N.J.:** Schering Corporation; PEG-Intron (peginterferon alfa-2b) package insert. October 2003.

10.**Wang Q, Miyakawa Y, Fox N, Kaushansky K.** Interferon-alpha directly represses megakaryopoiesis by inhibiting thrombopoietin-induced signaling through induction of SOCS-1. *Blood* 2000; 96:2093-2099.

11.**Ganser A, Carlo-Stella C, Greher J, Völkers B, Hoelzer D.** Effect of recombinant interferons alpha and gamma on human bone marrow-derived megakaryocytic progenitor cells. *Blood* 1987; 70:1173-1179.

12. **Dukes PP, Izadi P, Jorge OA, Shore NA, Gomperts E.** Inhibitory effects of interferon on mouse megakaryocytic progenitor cells in culture. *Exp Hematol* 1980; 8:1048-1056.

13. **Mazur EM, Richtsmeier WJ, South K.** Alpha-interferon: differential suppression of colony growth from human erythroid, myeloid, and megakaryocytic hematopoietic progenitor cells. *J Interferon Res* 1986; 6:199-206.

14.**Sata M, Yano Y, Yoshiyama Y, et al.** Mechanisms of thrombocytopenia induced by interferon therapy for chronic hepatitis B. *J Gastroenterol* 1997; 32:206-210.

15. **Dourakis SP, Deutsch M, Hadziyannis SJ.** Immune thrombocytopenia and alpha-interferon therapy. *J Hepatol* 1996; 25:972-975.

16. **Elefsiniotis IS, Pantazis KD, Fotos NV, Moulakakis A, Mavrogiannis C.** Late onset autoimmune thrombocytopenia associated with pegylated interferon-α-2b plus ribavirin treatment for chronic hepatitis C. *J Gastroenterol Hepatol* 2006; 21:622-623.

17. **Dormann H, Krebs S, Muth-Selbach U, et al.** Rapid onset of hematotoxic effects after interferon alpha in hepatitis C. *J Hepatol* 2000; 32:1041-1042.

18.**Rustgi VK, Lee P, Finnegan S, Ershler W.** Safety and efficacy of recombinant human IL-11 (oprelvekin) in combination with interferon/ ribavirin in hepatitis C patients with thrombocytopenia. Hepatology 2002; 36(4 Pt 2):361A. Abstract.

19. **Mayet WJ, Hess G, Gerken G, Rossol S, Voth R, Manns M, Meyer-zum-Buschenfelde KH.** Treatment of chronic type B hepatitis with recombinant alpha-

interferon induces autoantibodies not specific for autoimmune chronic hepatitis. Hepatology 1989; 10:24-8.

20. **Preziati D, La Rosa L, Covini G, Marcelli R, Rescalli S, Persani L, Del Ninno E, Meroni PL, Colombo M, Beck-Peccoz P.** Autoimmunity and thyroid function in patients with chronic active hepatitis treated with recombinant interferon alpha-2a. Eur J Endocrinol 1995;132:587-93.

21. **Carella C, Amato G, Biondi B, Rotondi M, Morisco F, Tuccillo C, Chiuchiolo N, Signoriello G, Caporaso N, Lombardi G.** Longitudinal study of antibodies against thyroid in patients undergoing interferon-a therapy for HCV chronic hepatitis. Horm Res 1995; 44:110-4.

22. **Marcellin P, Pouteau M, Renard P, Grynblat J-M, Colas Linhart N, Bardet P, Bok B, Benhamou J-P.** Sustained hypothyroidism induced by recombinant a interferon in patients with chronic hepatitis C. Gut 1992; 33:855-6.

23. **Noda K, Enomoto N, Arai K, Masuda E, Yamada Y, Suzuki K, Tanaka M, Yoshihara H.** Induction of antinuclear antibody after interferon therapy in patients with type-C chronic hepatitis: its relation to the efficacy oftherapy. Scand J Gastroenterol 1996; 31:716-22.

24. **Nagayama Y, Ohta K, Tsuruta M, Takeshita A, Kimura H, Hamasaki K, Ashizawa K, Nakata K, Yokoyama N, Nagataki S.** Exacerbation of thyroid autoimmunity by interferon alpha treatment in patients with chronic viral hepatitis: our studies and review of the literature. Endocr J 1994; 41:565-72.

25. **Imagawa A, Itoh N, Hanafusa T, Oda Y, Waguri M, Miyagawa J-l, Kono N, Kuwajima M, Matsuzawa Y.** Autoimmune endocrine disease induced by recombinant interferon-a therapy for chronic active type C hepatitis. J Clin Endocrinol Metab 1995; 80:922 6.

26. **Lisker-Melman M, Di Bisceglie AM, Usala SJ, Weintraub B, Murray LM, Hoofnagle JH.** Development of thyroid disease during therapy of chronic viral hepatitis with interferon alfa. Gastroenterology 1992; 102:2155-60.

27. **Marazuela M, Garcia-Buey L, Gonzalez-Fernandez B, Garcia-Monzon C, Arranz A, Borque MJ, Moreno-Otero R.** Thyroid autoimmune disorders in

patients with chronic hepatitis C before and during interferon-a therapy. Clin Endocrinol (Oxf) 1996;44:635-42.

28. Baudin E, Marcellin P, Pouteau M, Colas-Linhart N, Le Floch J-P, Lemmonier C, Benhamou J-P, Bok B. Reversibility of thyroid dysfunction induced by recombinant alpha interferon in chronic hepatitis C. Clin Endocrinol(Oxf) 1993;39:657-61.

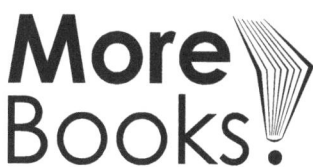

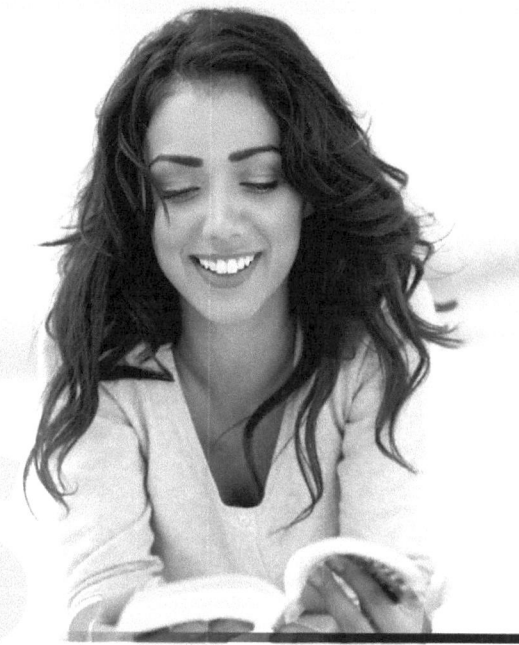

i want morebooks!

Buy your books fast and straightforward online - at one of world's fastest growing online book stores! Environmentally sound due to Print-on-Demand technologies.

Buy your books online at
www.get-morebooks.com

Kaufen Sie Ihre Bücher schnell und unkompliziert online – auf einer der am schnellsten wachsenden Buchhandelsplattformen weltweit! Dank Print-On-Demand umwelt- und ressourcenschonend produziert.

Bücher schneller online kaufen
www.morebooks.de

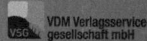 VDM Verlagsservicegesellschaft mbH
Heinrich-Böcking-Str. 6-8   Telefon: +49 681 3720 174   info@vdm-vsg.de
D - 66121 Saarbrücken   Telefax: +49 681 3720 1749   www.vdm-vsg.de

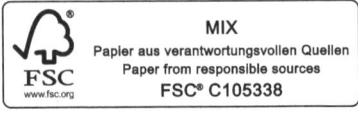

Printed by Books on Demand GmbH, Norderstedt / Germany